"This is a delightful, easy-to-follow guide for today's busy woman. Fern leads you through a complete workout and also offers terrific motivating tips to look and feel good."

Marci Shimoff, co-author *Chicken Soup for the Woman's Soul*

"Fern has developed an answer to the fitness equation of good nutrition and enjoyable exercise. Her advice is based on what works and what fits into our busy lives. The benefits of following Fern's advice are well worth the effort. You'll feel better, look better, and have more energy to enjoy life."

Sheah Rarbach, M.S., R.D., L.D., Nutritionist

"Fern has created the compact essential primer for those on the go with minimum of time to exercise. She provides maximum inspiration and all around tips for healthfulness."

Linda Marraccini, M.D., ABFP
Past President, Florida Academy of Family Physicians

"Fern is a fine professional as well as a delightful person. She has maintained my fitness program and proper nutritional regimen for the past 14 years. I actually look and feel better now than I did when I was years younger."

Toby Lerner Ansin, founder, Miami City Ballet

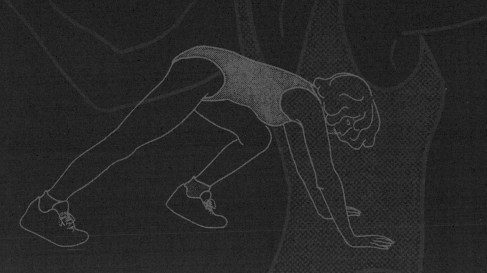

How to Be

Your Own
Personal Trainer

ON THE ROAD AND AT HOME

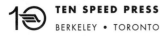

TEN SPEED PRESS
BERKELEY • TORONTO

Fern Starr

Ten Speed Press
Box 7123
Berkeley, California 94707
www.tenspeed.com

Distributed in Australia by Simon & Schuster Australia, in Canada by
Ten Speed Press Canada, in New Zealand by Southern Publishers Group,
in South Africa by Real Books, in Southeast Asia by Berkeley Books, and
in the United Kingdom and Europe by Airlift Books.

Cover and book design: Sandy Drooker
Illustrations: Laura Southworth

Library of Congress Cataloging-in-Publication Data on file with publisher

Printed in Canada
First printing, 2000

1 2 3 4 5 6 7 8 9 10 — 05 04 03 02 01 00

To my two loving daughters,
Teri and Laura

For helping make this book possible, I thank the following people for their time, caring, support, and assistance:

Cherie, Laura, David, Toby, Eva, Luis, Michello, Sharon, Lorraine, Mitchell, Steve, Susan, Patty, Matt, Gloria, Star, Carole, Courtney, and all the terrific people who have been my clients, allowing me, also, to learn from them.

Contents

My Dear Reader,

I wrote this book because so many of the people I've worked with asked me to please give them a guide they could follow.

The purpose of my book is to help you help yourself. I want to support and encourage you to look, feel, and be your best. This is a guide to making your workouts and healthy eating habits a permanent part of your lifestyle, with the same high priority you give to brushing your teeth.

My goal was to keep it simple. This is not a tedious text-book. It is an uncomplicated "how to" guide to get you in shape and feeling great, even with a minimal amount of time available.

Once you begin your program, you will discover it is the best way to handle and reduce stress and PMS. Researchers have found that working out can help avoid or reduce the symptoms of arthritis, osteoporosis, diabetes, heart disease, strokes, high blood pressure, and cancer.

I am constantly being asked, "Where do you get all that energy?" You too will find that the more you work out, the more energy you have.

I am an astute student of physical and mental health. I firmly believe there is a direct supportive relationship between mind and body. My simple, holistic approach to overall good health works through nonjudgmental, gentle, support-ive, honest, positive motivation, with emphasis on preven-tion, personal growth, and maintenance.

I am a University of Michigan graduate with 30 years of experience in the fitness and health fields. I've been a high-school physical education teacher and coach, competitive tennis player, marathon runner, and golfer. For the past 16 years I have been involved in personal training, nutrition counseling, and stress management. I have a great deal of experience with (and compassion for) people and their needs.

This is basically a no equipment program, although at home you will need a set of 3-lb. and/or 5-lb. weights. Your rou-tine will include a mild warm-up and stretching, a cardiovascular workout (maintaining a comfortably elevated heart rate), weight-bearing and strength-training moves, abdominals, stretching, and yoga.

The beauty of this complete routine is you can do it "on the road" without any equipment, in the privacy of your own room. You will benefit from as little as 15 minutes a day— though it's great if you can build up to a half hour to an hour. I suggest you follow the order presented in the book. Working the larger muscles first avoids fatigue; alternating upper- and lower-body work gives each set of muscles time to rest and recover. Cooling down with stretching and many yoga positions helps you to maintain and increase youthful flexibility, avoid injury, and achieve mental serenity.

Throughout the book, you'll find quick healthy lifestyle tips to keep you motivated. Finally, there's a Beautiful Body Journal, a simple method of behavior modification to help you become aware of and modify your eating and drinking habits.

I urge you to make this commitment to yourself. No one else can do it for you. By opening this book, you have already taken the first step. Read on, and enjoy your new feelings of health, strength, and well-being.

Love,

Fern

A workout is 25 percent perspiration and **75 percent determination**—it is one part physical exertion and three parts self-discipline.

A workout makes you better today than you were yesterday. It strengthens your body, relaxes your mind, and bolsters your spirit.

A workout is a form of rebirth. When you finish a good workout, you don't simply feel better, you feel better about yourself.

A workout is a wise use of time and an **investment in excellence**. It is a personal triumph over laziness and procrastination.

A workout is the badge of a winner—it identifies you as organized, goal-oriented, **in charge of your destiny**.

Improving your **appearance and well-being** is part of your overall life strategy. Focus on how you look **and** how you feel.

List the reasons you have decided to work out:

1. _____

2. _____

3. _____

4. _____

5. _____

List the benefits you will derive from working out:

1. _____

2. _____

3. _____

4. _____

5. _____

Write your short-term goals:

(for example, lose 1/2 to 1 pound a week, firm/sculpt body, reduce stress, have more energy)

1. _____

2. _____

3. _____

4. _____

5. _____

Write your long-term goals:

(for example, lose 3 inches around waist, lose 15 pounds, improve stamina, gain a more positive attitude)

1. _____

2. _____

3. _____

4. _____

5. _____

If you have difficulty staying motivated:

- First, read through the whole book
- Make a commitment to working out regularly for three months.
- Mornings are best—as the day progresses, time runs out.
- Rise just 15 to 30 minutes earlier.
- Work out first thing on rising—don't even think about looking at the paper or making a phone call. Consider taking the phone off the hook or just don't answer it.
- You do not need to do everything in this book. Start with just 10 or 15 minutes of the cardiovascular workouts, two or three times a week. As you increase your stamina, add to your routine.

- Do your strength training at a different time (perhaps the end of the day, while watching TV).
- If you have a setback, it's OK (we all do). Just start again and take 1 workout at a time.
- DON'T TELL ANYONE. Enjoy people noticing how good you look.
- Write in your Beautiful Body Journal every day—even when you have a temporary lapse in your new program. It's all part of your journey.
- Your journal is your private business. You need not share it with anyone; just enjoy your progress.

18 Consult with your physician before starting your workout program.

Some terms explained

- A rep (repetition) is 1 count.
- A set is a number of reps.
- "3 sets" means do 10 reps . . . rest 1 minute . . . do 2 more sets of 10 reps resting 1 minute between sets.

Warming Up

For mild stretching, warming up, and working the waist. At home, use a broom handle. On the road, use a towel or a tie.

Pole swings #1

Stand with feet shoulder width apart. Place pole behind neck, extending arms wide, knees flexed. Turn body from the hips only. Let head move with body turn.

20 reps (10 turns to both sides).

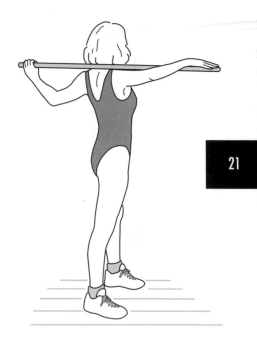

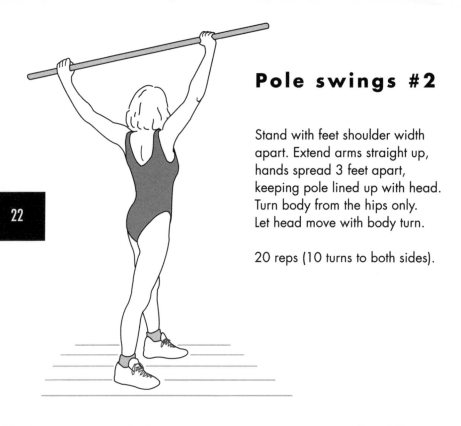

Pole swings #2

Stand with feet shoulder width apart. Extend arms straight up, hands spread 3 feet apart, keeping pole lined up with head. Turn body from the hips only. Let head move with body turn.

20 reps (10 turns to both sides).

Pole swings #3

Stand with feet shoulder width apart. Extend arms straight up, hands 3 feet apart. Standing up tall, knees flexed, bend to the side, trying to touch end of pole to the side of your leg. Go as far as a comfortable stretch only, pause, then turn to the other side.

20 reps (10 turns to both sides).

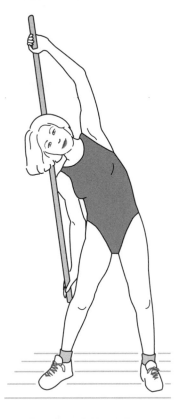

Pole swings (advanced)

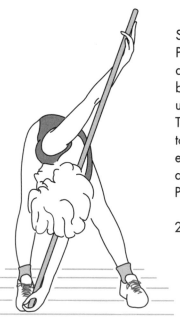

Stand with feet 2 feet apart. Pole behind head, hands 3 feet apart, knees flexed. Bend upper body over from waist, bringing upper body close to lower body. Turn at the waist, allowing head to turn with body. Try to point end of pole to opposite foot—go as far as a comfortable stretch. Pause and turn to other side.

20 reps (10 reps to both sides).

Standing oblique side bends

This move helps to sculpt the waist.

Holding a 3-lb. or 5-lb. weight, slowly slide down side of leg, keeping shoulder aligned with knee.

10 reps. Repeat on other side. 2 sets each side.

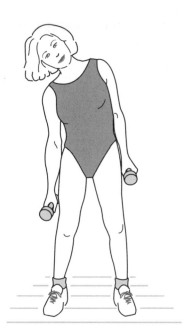

If you want to raise your metabolism and lose weight: GET PHYSICAL!

- Walk instead of riding. Climbing steps is a cardiovascular workout. To work butt, climb double steps, landing on heels.
- Stand instead of sitting (stand when you are on the phone).
- Sit instead of lying down.

To lose weight:

- Change eating habits.
- Do a cardiovascular workout 5 times each week.
- Do strength training 3 times each week.

28 A cardiovascular workout is a physical activity that sustains an elevated heart rate.

You can determine your training heart rate with this formula:

Subtract your age from 220, then multiply by 0.60 or 0.65. For example: 220 – 40 = 180 x 0.60 = 108 beats per minute; 220 – 40 = 180 x 0.65 = 117 beats per minute.

- A cardiovascular workout often decreases your appetite and enhances your mood and energy level.
- Do your cardiovascular workout first to warm the muscles and prevent injury.
- A cardiovascular workout aids in the treatment of diabetes. With a doctor's supervision, some have lowered or even eliminated insulin medication by combining workouts with healthy eating habits.
- Exercise helps relieve arthritis because it aids in maintaining ideal body weight. (Proper mild stretching increases flexibility.)

Cardiovascular Workouts

weight-bearing

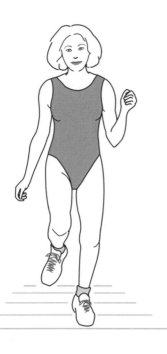

March in place, swinging arms at sides

Variations:
- Go forward and backward.
- Raise knees higher for more exertion.

To work your gluteals (butt), squeeze tight on each step. Try playing upbeat music, or watching TV.

15–30 minutes.

Hand runs

This is a real workout! Build up to more reps slowly—don't overdo it.

Place hands on the floor with bent knees, weight on hands. Run feet forward and backward. Count each step; increase number as stamina improves.

Start with 25 reps; gradually work up to 300–500 reps.

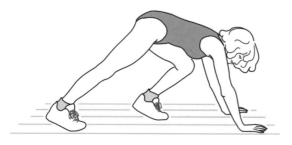

Hand jumps

Place hands on floor with bent knees, weight on hands, feet together. Take small jumps forward and back, 1 count for each jump.

Start with 20 reps; work up to 50–100 reps.

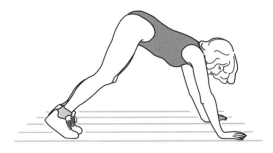

Hand twist jumps

Place hands on floor with bent knees, weight on hands, feet together. Do small twist jumps, turning your feet right and left, in place, 1 count for each twist jump.

Start with 20 reps; work up to 50–100 reps.

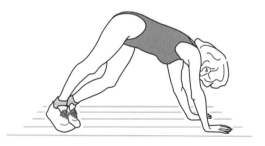

Hand high kicks

Try this advanced move once you've mastered the hand runs and jumps.

Place hands on floor with bent knees, weight on hands. With a fast pace, high kick behind you, alternating feet, 1 count for each step.

Start with 20 reps, work up to 100 reps.

Self-love is making a commitment to a fitness lifestyle.

38 Take up new interests that are not sedentary.

It is empowering to improve your physical appearance.

BREATHE

Your body needs oxygen to function at its best. Inhale through your nose, exhale through your mouth. Just remember, **"exhale on the exertion."** Avoid holding your breath—this raises blood pressure and increases fatigue.

Upper Body

weight resistance

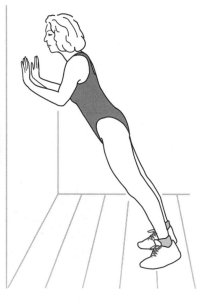

Wall push-offs

These work the pectorals and biceps.

Stand in front of wall, arms fully extended. Place palms against wall at chest height, shoulder width apart. Keeping body straight (with no hip movement), bend elbows, bringing forehead to wall. Exhale through mouth as you push away.

Work up to 20 reps.

Corner wall push-offs

These both work and stretch the pectorals.

Face a corner and place palms against walls at chest height, keeping body straight. Bend elbows, bringing body towards corner. Go as far as a comfortable stretch only.

10 reps.

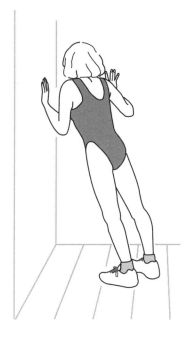

Modified push-ups

A workout for pectorals and biceps.

On hands and knees, cross ankles, supporting all your weight on straight arms, hands slightly wider than shoulder width apart. Bend arms to bring thighs to floor. Exhale through mouth as you push up.

Work up to 20 reps.

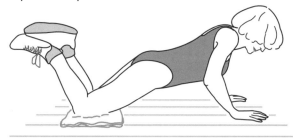

Full body push-ups

A more demanding workout for pectorals and biceps.

Support yourself on palms and balls of feet. Bend elbows and lower body, attempting to touch chest to floor. Keep body straight; avoid letting hips arch up or sag. Exhale through mouth as you push up.

Work up to 20 reps.

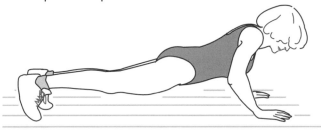

Chair dip

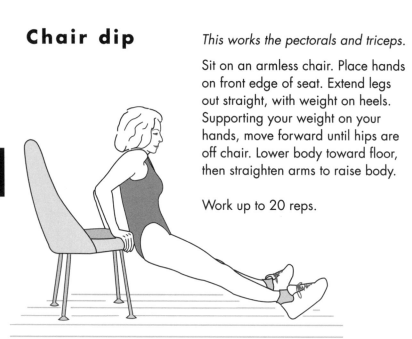

This works the pectorals and triceps.

Sit on an armless chair. Place hands on front edge of seat. Extend legs out straight, with weight on heels. Supporting your weight on your hands, move forward until hips are off chair. Lower body toward floor, then straighten arms to raise body.

Work up to 20 reps.

Keep your body as young, fit, and flexible as your mind.

Taking charge of your body is sometimes the first step in **taking charge of your life**.

Lower Body

let's work those legs!

Have a seat!

Works the quadriceps to support knees and strengthen legs.

Stand against wall or door, leaning on heels, back of head and torso against wall. Slide down wall, walking on heels away from door until thighs are parallel to the floor. Hold and count— work up to 100.

Lunge

*(**Caution:** avoid this exercise if you have knee problems.) Works the quadriceps, gluteals, and hamstrings.*

Stand with feet together, knees lined up with toes. Take a long step forward onto heel, bending back knee toward floor. Don't allow front knee to extend beyond front of ankle. Return to starting position.

10 reps with 1 leg, then 10 reps with the other. Work up to 3 sets for each leg. To increase intensity, hold hand weights.

Walking lunges

Try this advanced move once you've mastered standing lunges.

Same as lunges, only lunge across the room taking giant steps. To increase intensity, hold hand weights.

Back lunges

This variation works the gluteals.
Stand with feet together. Step
backward, lowering that knee
toward the floor. Return to starting position. 10 reps with 1 leg,
then 10 reps with the other.
Work up to 3 sets for each leg.
To increase intensity, hold hand
weights.

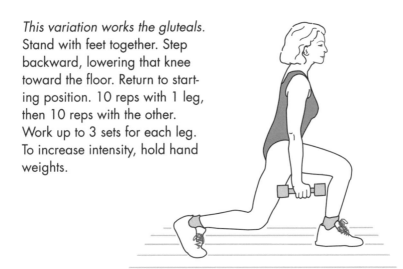

Squats

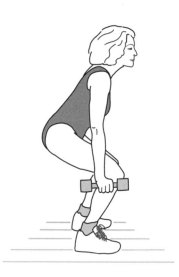

These work the hamstrings, quadriceps, and gluteals.

Pretend you are standing in front of a chair. Place feet shoulder width apart, with weight on heels. Bend knees and pretend to sit down. Try to get thighs parallel to floor. Pause, tighten butt, and **slowly** straighten back up. On last rep of each set, hold seated position for 10 seconds. Hold hand weights to increase intensity.

10 reps; work up to 3 sets.

Side lunge

Works the upper body and thighs.

Stand with feet together. Hold a 3-lb. or 5-lb. weight with both hands, close to your chest. With right leg, take a wide step to the side, bending knee (keep left leg straight, feeling stretch on inner thigh). As you step to the side, push the weight forward (chest high) by straightening arms. Then return to starting position with weight close to chest, feet together. Repeat to left side.

10 reps; work up to three sets.

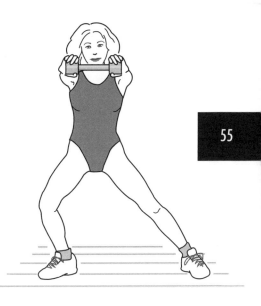

Leg extensions
(strengthen those knees!)

These target the quadriceps to maintain strong, healthy knees. I recommend you start with just the weight of shoes. When you can do 3 sets of 10 reps, add 5-lb. ankle weights.

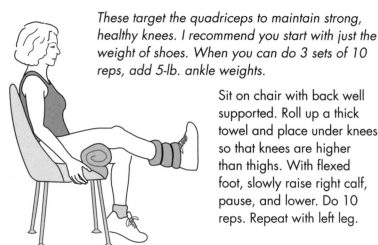

Sit on chair with back well supported. Roll up a thick towel and place under knees so that knees are higher than thighs. With flexed foot, slowly raise right calf, pause, and lower. Do 10 reps. Repeat with left leg.

10 reps each leg; work up to 3 sets.

Age is an attitude—become **ageless**.

Schedule your daily workout in your appointment calendar. Writing is a commit-ment—make your workout a high priority.

You do not have time to **not** work out.

Avoid injury: listen to your body. If you feel pain—STOP. Lighter weights and more repetitions will help avoid injury. Increase intensity slowly; allow at least 1 week for each increase.

WEIGHT TRAINING

I recommend that you begin with lighter weights and more repetitions to avoid injury. You may want to begin your program with 2-lb. or 3-lb. weights; work your way up to 5-lb. weights. You are using enough weight if you feel some resistance and muscle fatigue at the end of a set (of 10 reps).

WEIGHT SUBSTITUTES

When you are on the road, you can fill plastic
1.5 L bottles with water (about 4 lbs.). (Always
carry bottled water to drink on the road; you will
feel better and it even inhibits the appetite!) You
can also use books, shoes, rocks—be creative!
Or train without weights and tighten the muscles
that you are working.

Weight Training

seated

Seated, bent-over laterals

An aid to good posture, this exercise works the deltoids (shoulders) and trapezius (back muscle).

Sit with feet 1 foot apart, holding 3-lb. or 5-lb. weights. Bend over so your upper body is supported by your thighs. Exhale and slowly lift weights to the side, to shoulder height. Pause, inhale, and slowly lower weights to starting position.

10 reps, 2 or 3 sets.

Seated bent-over lifts

Works the trapezius and triceps.

Sit with feet 1 foot apart, holding 3-lb. or 5-lb. weights. Bend over so your upper body is supported by your thighs. Extend arms down toward the floor, palms facing backward. Exhale and bend elbows, lifting weights, squeezing shoulder blades together, and turning hands so that palms face forward. Then inhale and return weights to starting position.

10 reps, 2 or 3 sets.

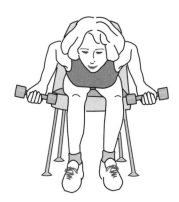

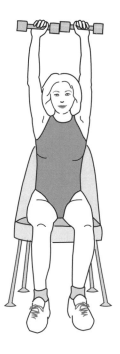

Seated overhead press

Works the trapezius, triceps, and deltoids.

Sit in a chair, with your back well supported. Hold 3-lb. or 5-lb. weights at shoulder height with arms close to body, palms facing each other. Exhaling, raise and extend arms fully, with weights lined up with back of head. Turn hands so that ends of weights touch. Inhale and lower weights to starting position.

10 reps, 2 or 3 sets.

Biceps curl

Better than spinach for your 'Popeye' muscles.

Sit holding 3-lb. or 5-lb. weights. Pressing backs of upper arms against body, alternate lifting weights by bending elbows and flexing biceps.

10 reps each arm; 2 or 3 sets.

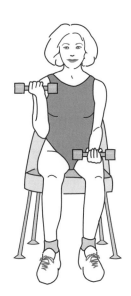

If you keep doing what you always did, you will keep getting what you always got!!!

There's a bad virus going around—it's called **"excusitis."**

When you are **numero uno**, no excuse is acceptable because **you** are high priority. Do not think—**Do it!**

You are good at problem-solving. Getting in shape is problem-solving.

Abdominals

These exercises tighten and strengthen for a more fit appearance, and help support your back. (To spot-reduce, do cardiovascular workouts and change your eating and drinking habits.)

Abdominals

This one's a great "de-stresser."

Lie on back, knees bent. Inhale, inflating stomach. Then exhale, pressing lower back into floor, tightening and hollowing abdomen, and tightening butt. Feel as if you're pressing your stomach into the floor; hold.

10 reps.

You can do this seated, too—in your car, at the office, any time you feel **stressed out**.

Abdominal Crunches

Lie on back, knees bent, feet on floor. Cross arms in an X behind your head so that head and neck are supported, with hands loose. Press lower back into floor and inhale through nose. Press down and tighten lower abdomen. Exhale through mouth and lift shoulder blades 2–3 inches off floor. Pause and slowly return to starting position.

20 reps; work up to 2 sets of 50.

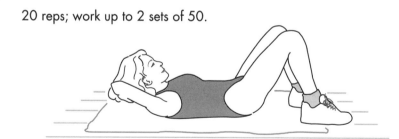

Abdominals

This move works the obliques and sculpts your waist.

Lie on back. Bend right knee and cross left leg over right thigh. Place right hand loosely behind head. Keeping elbow back, with tight abdomen, exhale through mouth and lift body, bringing right armpit toward left side. Pause in curled position, then return to starting position.

20 reps on 1 side; repeat on other side.

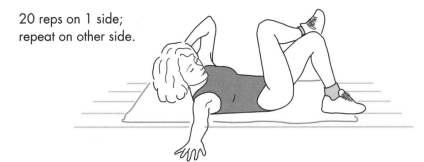

Unless you do strength training and weight-bearing exercise regularly, after age 25 you will lose up to 1/2 lb. of muscle every year.

Strength training (using body weight and/or weights) plays a major role in improving your physical appearance by **increasing muscle tissue.** You can weigh the same amount but have a firmer, leaner appearance.

78 Increase intensity slowly, allowing at least 1 week for each increase.

Increasing muscle tissue raises your **metabolism.** Loss of muscle tissue lowers your metabolism 1/2 percent every year, with an **increase in body fat.**

Strength training greatly reduces the risk of injury. It improves balance and strength. By stressing the bones (strengthening the skeletal system) it is a great aid in preventing and handling **osteoporosis**.

Beginners who did strength training regularly for just 2 months have gained 2 to 4 lbs. of muscle and increased their strength by 20 to 40 percent.

Weight Training

floor

Flies

These work the pectorals.

Lie on back, knees bent, lower back pressed to floor. Holding 3-lb. or 5-lb. weights, extend arms out to the side, lined up with shoulders. With elbows slightly flexed, raise weights over chest, keeping palms facing each other. Return to starting position.

10 reps; work up to 3 sets.

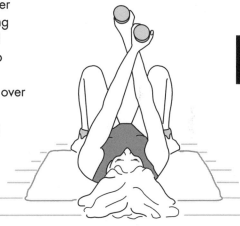

Triceps

This move really sculpts the backs of your upper arms.

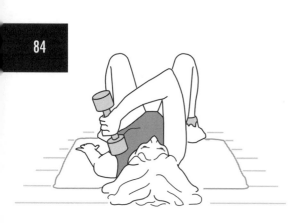

Lie on back, knees bent. Hold a 3-lb. or 5-lb. weight in right hand, resting on your left shoulder, palm facing feet. Raise arm, keeping elbow pointing to ceiling. Keep hand and elbow lined up with shoulders. Turn face to right side. Straighten your arm, moving forearm only and keeping upper arm still. Feel the triceps flexing. Return to starting position. 10 reps. Repeat with left arm. Work up to 3 sets for each arm.

Triceps extensions

Lie on back, knees bent, lower back pressed to floor. With both hands palms upward, grasp the ends of a 5-lb. or 10-lb. weight just above your head. Raise your bent upper arms to vertical (with weight above your forehead), then move your forearms to straighten arms and work the triceps. Return to starting position. 10 reps; work up to 3 sets. Begin with a 5-lb. weight and work up to a 10-lb.

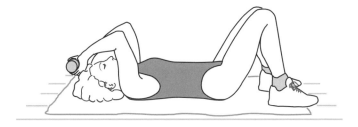

Overhead pullover

Works the latissimus (back) and deltoid (shoulder) muscles.

Lie on back, knees bent, lower back pressed to floor. Grasp one 5-lb. weight in both hands, over abdomen. Extend arms fully back over your head, bringing weight to floor. Then swing straight arms forward, bringing weight to abdomen.

10 reps; work up to 3 sets. Begin with a 5-lb. weight and work up to a 10-lb.

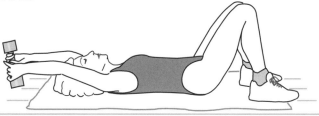

Presses

Works the triceps and pectorals.

Lie on back, knees bent, lower
back pressed to floor. Hold 3-lb.
or 5-lb. weights above chest,
palms facing each other. With
arms close to body, extend arms
fully upward, keeping weights
over chest and turning weights
so ends touch. Lower to starting
position.

10 reps; work up to 3 sets.

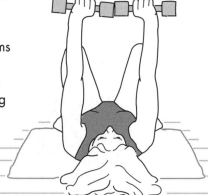

Stretching

- Stretching will increase your flexibility.
- Stretching will prevent most of the muscle soreness that often follows physical exertion.
- Stretching will aid in preventing many injuries.
- Do a warm-up before your workout; do stretching after your workout.
- Unless otherwise indicated, hold most stretches for 20 to 30 seconds.
- If you have back or neck problems, check these exercises with your doctor first.

Shoulder, neck, spine, hip stretch

Lie on back with arms out to the side, lined up with shoulders. Keep shoulders against the floor. Extend your straight right leg on floor. Bend your left leg and bring left knee over right leg, keeping left shoulder to floor. Bend right knee to side and straighten left leg to side (holding with right hand). Turn head, looking to the left. Hold. Repeat on other side.

Hamstring stretch

These help prevent the back injuries that often stem from tight hamstrings.

Lie on back with 1 leg bent, the other leg extended straight up, holding calf with one hand, pressing knee with your other. If you cannot straighten leg, wrap towel around calf. Hold 2 to 3 minutes. Repeat with other leg.

Hamstring stretch

Lie on back by a doorway.
Extend 1 leg through doorway.
Extend other leg upward against
wall, getting butt as close to wall
as possible. Hold 2 to 3 minutes.
Repeat with other leg.

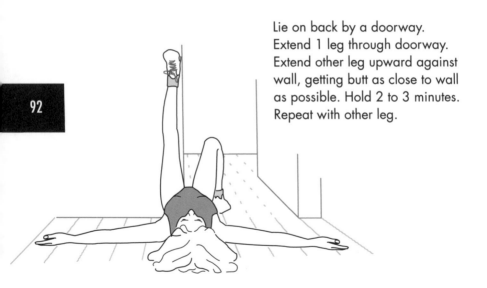

Inner thigh and hip stretch

Lie on back with legs raised together toward ceiling. Lower legs
out to the side, pushing calves outward with hands. Hold.
Optional: to work abdominals, raise head off floor.

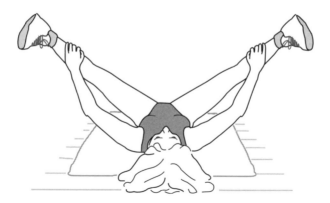

Hip and waist stretch

Lie on back, bending knees to chest. Extend arms to sides at shoulder height, keeping shoulders anchored to floor. Roll knees to side, trying to touch hip to floor. Turn head to opposite side. Hold.

10 reps each side.

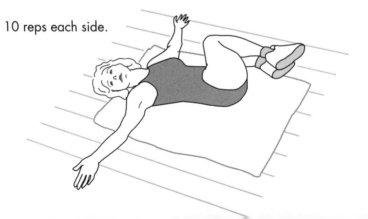

The spinal twist

Sit and extend left leg. Bend right leg and cross right foot over left thigh. Hold outside of left knee with left hand. Rest your weight on right hand on the floor behind you. Turn head and look over right shoulder. Hold 15 to 30 seconds. Repeat on other side.

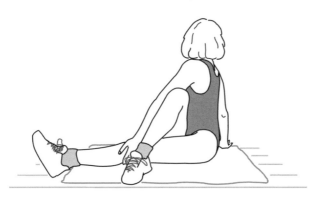

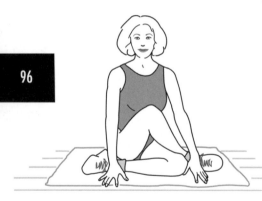

The pretzel

A great hip stretch!

Sit and cross legs, with right calf on top of left thigh, feet lined up away from butt. Place hands on floor forward of legs. Sit tall, trying to keep both sides of your butt as close to the floor as possible. Then sit tall. Hold 15 seconds. Repeat on other side.

Back Stretching
& Strengthening

Lower-back stretch

Lie on back.
1. Squeeze both knees to chest. Hold.
2. Extend 1 leg on floor and squeeze other knee to chest. Hold.
3. Repeat with other leg. Hold.

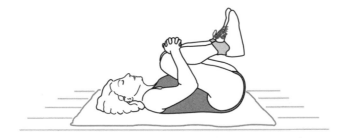

Opposite arm & leg extensions

A good back strengthener.

Lie on stomach, arms extended over head. Lift right arm and left leg, then lift left arm and right leg. 20 reps. Keeping arms and legs on floor, stretch right arm and left leg, then left arm and right leg. 20 reps.

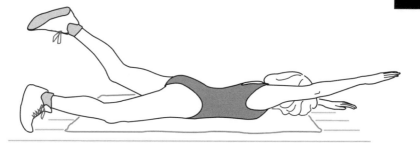

Back extensions

These target the lower back muscles.

Lie on stomach and place palms on the floor near shoulders. Contract lower back muscles and lift chest without using arms for support. Hold.

10 reps.

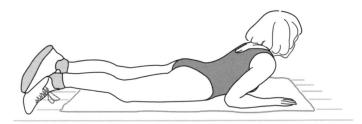

Scared cat

On hands and knees, keeping arms straight, arch back up. Hollow abdomen and tuck chin into neck. Hold. Flatten back, keeping arms straight, and tip head back. Hold. 3 reps.

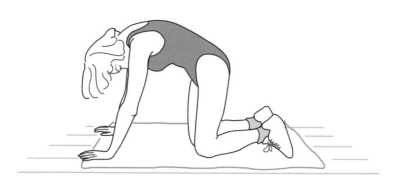

Sleeping baby

Kneel and let your body relax forward, forehead on floor, arms extended over head. Hold 15 seconds. Then slide arms down to your sides, palms up, eyes closed. Allow shoulders, arms, and hips to drop, totally "letting go." Stay in this position and mellow out.

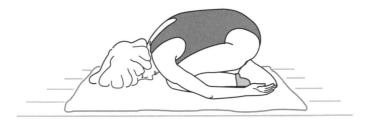

Hang loose

Sit on the edge of a chair. Bend upper body toward floor, armpits resting on legs, allowing head and arms to "hang loose." Totally let go for 2 to 3 minutes.

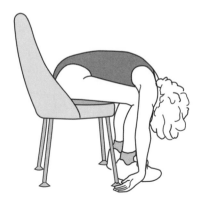

The turtle

With feet shoulder width apart, squat close to the floor, keeping heels to floor, arms inside knees, head hanging. Hold 30 seconds.

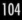

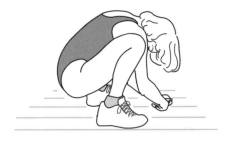

Standing Shoulder Stretches

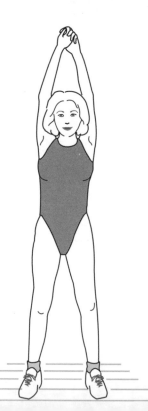

Raise arms and fully extend them overhead. Twist hands so right palm faces right and left palm faces left; interlace fingers. Keeping arms straight, pull back with shoulders. Hold.

3 reps.

Raise left arm and bend elbow with forearm behind head. Hold left elbow with right hand; gently pull and hold. Repeat on right arm. Hold 15 seconds.

3 reps each arm.

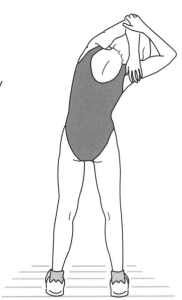

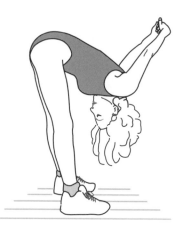

Interlace fingers behind back, draw elbows in, and raise arms. Slowly bend forward, bringing head toward knees. Keeping arms straight, bring hands forward toward head. Hold. Bending knees, slowly return to starting position.

Stand tall!

Stand with back to door. Raise arms so that back of hands, back of head, and heels are touching door. Keeping heels on floor, slide hands up high as you can, then press shoulders to door. Hold 10 seconds.

3 reps.

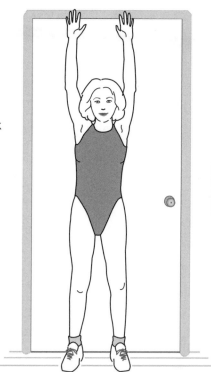

Neck Stretches

floor

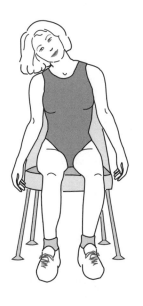

De-stress that neck!

Relax lower back and drop shoulders. Bend neck to the side, bringing ear toward shoulder. Hold 10 seconds. Repeat on other side.

3 reps on each side.

Relax lower back and drop head forward, chin toward neck. Place interlaced fingers on back of head and gently press head downward. Hold 20 seconds.

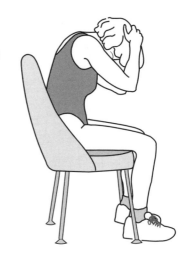

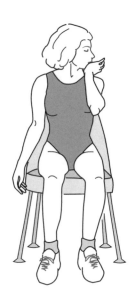

Relax lower back. Drop your chin and turn it toward left shoulder. Place palm of left hand on right side of chin and gently press toward left shoulder. Hold 10 seconds. Repeat on other side (right hand pressing left side of chin toward right shoulder).

3 reps on each side.

113

- Relax lower back. Make big slow circles with your shoulders from front to back.

- Squeeze upper back against back of neck.

- Then let head, shoulders, and arms drop, letting go.

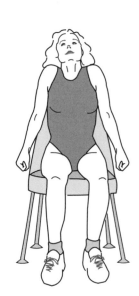

Now a big smile because you feel so much better!

Standing Stretches

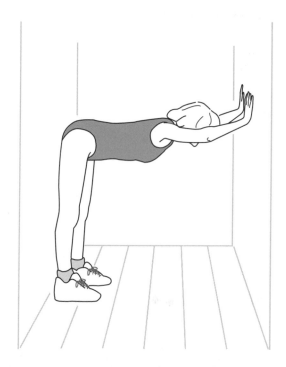

Extend arms against a wall, making an L shape with your body. Keeping heels on floor, push hips upward. Hold 20 seconds. Keeping heels on floor, bend both knees toward wall. Hold 20 seconds.

With 1 foot forward, **bend your back knee**, keeping both heels flat on the floor. Hold 20 seconds. Repeat on other side.

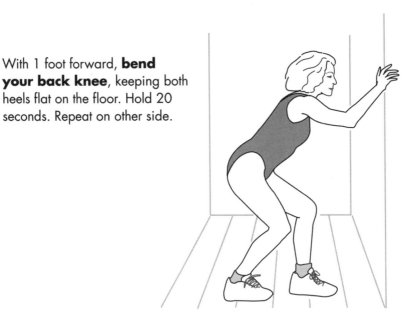

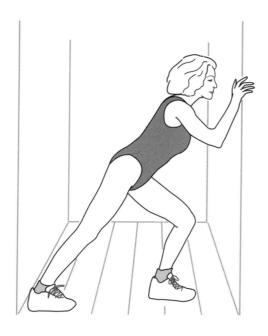

Slide 1 foot back, about a foot behind the other. Keeping back leg straight, **bend front knee forward**. Hold 20 seconds. Repeat on other side.

Stand sideways to a doorway molding. Line up ankle, hip, and shoulder to the molding. Reaching over your head with the far arm, place both hands on molding, fingertips touching. Now walk hands down until you feel a good stretch. Keep feet flat on floor. Hold 20 seconds. Repeat on other side.

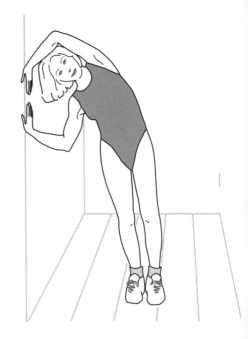

Standing Yoga Positions

The following yoga stretches will build your strength, balance, and flexibility.

You will also develop attractive, sculpted legs.

Tripod

With feet about a foot apart, line up heels at right angles—1 foot forward, 1 out to the side. Bend body over to that side; bringing it close to thigh. Don't force it; reach a comfortable stretch. Keep your lower arm close to your leg, the upper arm extended toward the ceiling. Turn head and look toward your raised hand. Hold 10 seconds. Repeat on other side.

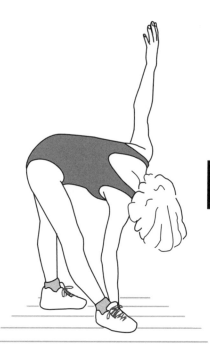

Downhill racer

This exercise helps develop balance. When you're first starting out, stand near a wall and place 2 fingers on it for support. It also helps to focus on a spot on the floor.

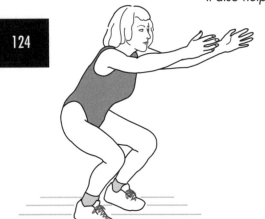

Stand with feet parallel, about a foot apart. Extend your arms forward at shoulder height. Keep shoulders and hands loose and soft.

1. With weight on heels, "sit down." Hold.
2. Rise up on toes and stand up. Hold.
3. Staying on toes, "sit down" again. Hold 10 to 30 seconds.

Soaring eagle

Keep focused on that spot on the floor!

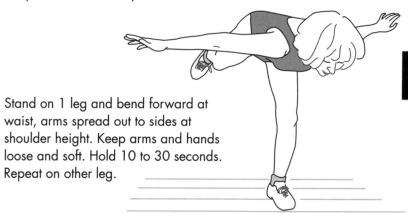

Stand on 1 leg and bend forward at
waist, arms spread out to sides at
shoulder height. Keep arms and hands
loose and soft. Hold 10 to 30 seconds.
Repeat on other leg.

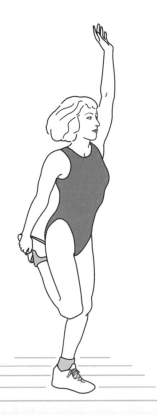

Flamingo

Stand on right leg. Bend left leg up behind you, holding foot with left hand. Keep knee close to right leg. Extend right arm toward ceiling. Advanced: rise up on toes. Hold 20 to 30 seconds. Repeat, standing on left leg.

In Your Face

A natural facelift! If you can laugh at yourself, do this in front of a mirror.

Open your mouth as wide as you can and stick your tongue out as far as possible (until you feel a strain). Open your eyes as wide as you can. Feel your neck and face straining. Hold 10 to 15 seconds.

3 reps.

It's easier to smile now because your face is so loose (and if you're looking in the mirror, you can't stop laughing).

Healthy Lifestyle Tips
to Raise Your Energy Level

- Exercise. It stimulates circulation and releases natural endorphins.
- Get enough sleep. You will function on a higher, calmer level. (Turn the TV off!)
- Do not skip meals. Include complex carbohydrates, protein, high fiber, low fat. Protein will sustain a high energy level. Snack on nonfat or light yogurt, a few nuts, an orange. Sugar creates an energy drop.
- Take small breaks—like a walk!
- Meditate for 15–20 minutes. Concentrate on your breathing only. Inhale, inflating stomach, hold 10 seconds. Then very slowly exhale through your mouth. Do 10 reps.

- Do something requiring your attention and concentration (cooking, sewing, playing a musical instrument, reading a book, taking a class, volunteer work, gardening). TV is passive and tiring.
- Take action. Resolve frustrating situations; they sap your energy.
- Naps are healthy. If you can, take a 20-minute nap.

Nurture yourself with good nutrition.

Increase your fiber intake to aid in weight loss. It makes you feel full and speeds up your metabolism because the body works harder to digest it.

132

High fiber will aid regularity. Be sure to have a substantial amount when you are "on the road."

Drink a minimum of 8 glasses of water every day.

Eat well to feel well.

Chew fresh parsley to clean your breath.

136 Working out regularly is often the first step in committing to healthy eating habits.

Smokers often find working out regularly is a **great incentive to quit smoking**.

Reward yourself. **Celebrate your successes, but not with food and drink**.

Tips for when you are "on the road," or "never have enough time"

- Plan ahead to avoid hunger attacks and eating empty calories.
- **Pack snacks in ziplock baggies**—fruit, baby carrots, microwaved small red potatoes, rice cakes, light yogurt, dry-roasted peanuts and raisin mix, bagels with natural peanut butter, bottled water.
- **Eat high-fiber, low-fat, live foods**—like fresh fruits and vegetables—instead of canned, processed, and packaged foods.
- Whole fresh fruit is better than fruit juice. You get the **fiber**—and it's more filling and satisfying.

- **Before going to cocktail parties** and late dinners, eat carrots, cantaloupe, rice cakes. You will then be able to resist those greasy hors d'oeuvres and other temptations that you would later regret that you ate because you were "famished."
- **A great meal to start or end the day:** Oatmeal (microwaved is fine), skim milk and fresh fruit.

To maintain regularity:

- Drink an 8-oz. glass of water when you arise; drink 8 to 10 glasses during the day.
- A high-fiber diet really works (2 salads a day with vinegar or nonfat dressing).
- Eat little or no refined sugar.
- Avoid cheese (low-fat cottage cheese is fine).
- Exercise.
- Do stress-reducing activities (stress is constipating).
- **LAUGH A LOT!** Develop a sense of humor.

Hydrate your **skin** and **body**. Drink lots of water. Drink before, during, and after working out.

High-fiber foods are satisfying and low in calories: baked potato (eat the skin) corn, beans, whole grains, brown rice, fruits, vegetables, salads.

Our bodies need *some* fat; I recommend 15–20 percent fat in your diet. However, avoid adding fat (butter or margarine, cream, oil), although a small amount of olive oil is fine. Low-fat or nonfat yogurt or cottage cheese goes well on a baked potato.

Get into the habit of reading labels.

Improving your physical appearance is **empowering**.

Be good to yourself. Exercise regularly, eat enjoyable healthy food, make **laughing a daily habit**, love and be lovable.

Find a picture of how you would like to look—
a magazine photo that resembles you. Post it
where you can look at it every morning and
every evening.

Your Beautiful Body Journal

Chart your progress:
- Enter your measurements now.
- Do not weigh yourself more than once a week.
- Pay more attention to how your clothes fit.
- Measure yourself once a month.

DATE						
RESTING PULSE						
WEIGHT						
BUST (FOR WOMEN)						
CHEST (FOR MEN)						
BUTT (WOMEN)						
WAIST						
HIPS						
UPPER THIGH						
UPPER ARM						

Each day:

- Record what you ate or drank and the time of day.
- Estimate the calories you consumed and total them.
- Record how you exercised and the length of time.
- You will appreciate looking back and seeing your progress.

EXAMPLE

Day: 1-1-99   **Calories**

07:00 AM	Oatmeal, cup skim milk, banana	250
10:00 AM	Light yogurt	100
01:00 PM	Turkey pita sandwich	350
03:00 PM	Apple	100
07:00 PM	Pasta, chicken breast, broccoli, salad	500
09:00 PM	Low-fat frozen yogurt	200

Workout: 1 hour fast walk and weight training   **Total:** 1500